# Voices of Strength and Hope
## for a friend with AIDS

By Joseph Gallagher

SHEED & WARD

Sheed & Ward ™ is a service of National Catholic Reporter Publishing, Inc.

Library of Congress Catalog Card Number: 87- 61464


ISBN: 1-55612-073-7


Published by:  Sheed & Ward
115 E. Armour Blvd., P.O. Box 414292
Kansas City, MO 64141-4292

To order, call: (800) 821-7926

## Dedication

*To my AIDS "buddy," Allen. After watching a TV special on AIDS he said to me: "The program didn't have much to offer to anybody who already has AIDS." Thank you, Allen of the gentle touch, for motivating me to write in your honor this well-wishing letter. I am thankful that your final good surprise on earth was a more easeful death than you expected. May all your brother and sister patients rejoice in their own good surprises.*

### Dear Friend with AIDS:

**I** presume to call you "friend," though I do not know you. But you are a brother or sister of mine in the human family, and you find yourself with a very heavy cross to bear. "I am Joseph, your brother," and I want to befriend you — just as I would want to be befriended in your stead.

Mainly, I want to comfort you, but with the kind of comfort that has a "fort" in it. As you may know, the word "comfort" originally meant to be "strong with" someone. I want to share with you some thoughts and voices that have brought needed strength to me and to others. May these words help convince you of your own resources and spur you to tap some of the enduring wells of fortitude discussed in these pages.

This letter contains quite a few of my favorite quotes, garnered through the years. If I could have found better words or ideas of my own, I would have used them. On this occasion, I want to share the best I've found, no matter whose voice is speaking.

Words, I know, are not everything. At times they are nothing or can seem even less than nothing. So I appreciate Shakespeare's warning against trying to "patch grief with proverbs." More recently, reflecting a down moment, Christopher Cross has sung, "All the words of wisdom, they never seem to ease the pain. All the words of wisdom sound the same."

I am acutely aware that there are events and situations

**1**

in life that are honored most decently by silence and by no trivializing or desecrating attempts to "explain."

Still, if "there is a time for keeping silence," there is also "a time for speaking." I can't doubt it: If the moment is ripe, words can strike like lightning and reveal by their energizing radiance a saving way out or a saving way through. At other times they can bring a sudden, soothing balm. I will be well rewarded if such is your experience even once as you ponder these pages.

## Some background

You don't know me, so I'd like to introduce myself. I'm in my 50s. I had a heart attack in 1979 and coronary bypass surgery in 1980. I still have coronary artery disease. More than the average person, I could be gathered to the bosom of my ancestors on short notice. In other words, like you, I am especially aware of death and of my own fragility.

Our comradeship on this score reminds me of two remarkable youngsters from Westernport, Md., whom I met six years ago. Michael Mertz and his older brother Francis both had terminal cancer. Scarcely a teenager, Michael said he wasn't afraid to die, so he would go first and smooth the way for Francis. Michael died Monday, Feb. 1, 1982. Francis died that Friday. (Now a healthy baby brother carries on their middle names.)

I was ordained a Catholic priest over 30 years ago and have enjoyed many unique opportunities to know all sorts of people with all sorts of problems. I hope I've helped some of them, but I know I've learned from many of them. What I've learned most, perhaps, is the wisdom of this old saying: "To know all is to forgive all." (If that's an exaggeration, it's the most creative and appropriate one an earthling can commit.)

Put another way:

*There's so much good in the worst of us*
*and so many faults in the best of us*

2

*that it makes no sense for any of us*
*to stand in judgment on the rest of us.*

Although I am a clergyman, I am talking to you now, with respect and modesty, simply and solely as one friend-needing, mistake-making, pain-fearing, death-bound human being to another. All I want is the privilege of sharing with you some road-tested attitudes toward adversity that have fortified me and others. Pardon me if some of the considerations don't apply to your situation.

I ask one favor: No matter what harsh things you may have heard about the Catholic church and some of its teachings and some of its spokesmen, please don't presume you automatically know my thoughts and feelings on controversial topics. Like the biblical Jacob wrestling with his angel, I and many another have grappled for long years with the actual or presumed teachings of the Bible, Christianity and the church.

Like any person striving to be conscientious, in the end I make up my own mind. Or as Father Rank says on the final page of Graham Greene's novel *The Heart of the Matter*, "The Church knows all the rules, but it doesn't know what goes on in a single human heart."

To put the matter in yet another way: As any other church member consciously or unconsciously does and must do, I decide for myself which religious teachings get priority treatment in my life.

As you might expect, I am a transfixed admirer of that brother human being of ours named Jesus Christ — the Jesus revealed in the Gospels and the Jesus reincarnated in brave, compassionate and saintly human beings who try to live out his teachings and manifest his spirit. I hear his voice, for instance, when I hear Mother Teresa of Calcutta saying, "AIDS victims are wanted, they are loved, and they will go home to God with pure hearts."

But when I hear a self-assured and judgmental spokesperson of any biblical religion talking about AIDS as God's vengeance on sin, (especially on little children, I suppose)

**3**

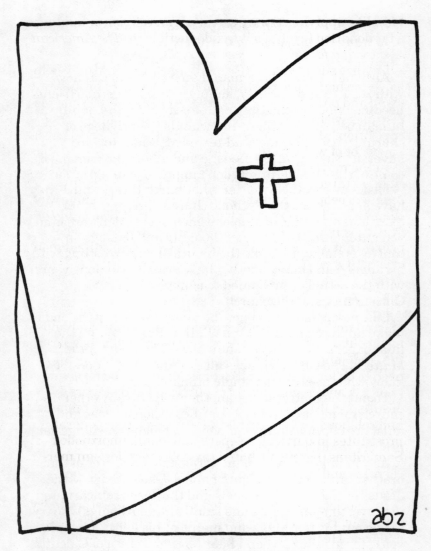

"The church knows all the rules, but it doesn't know what goes on in a single human heart."

I feel like applying to the nearest pagan religion or mailing a fat donation (even if not tax-deductible) to *The American Association for the Advancement of Atheism.*

I realize such a reaction is irrational and would only help leave the bigness of the Bible in hands that are pitifully small and pitifully unaware that they are small. (When his disciples wished to call down fire and brimstone on "the opposition," Jesus rebuked them with the words: "You know not of what spirit you are.")

In the movie *Buddies*, the man suffering from AIDS is right on target when he says, "The trouble with many religious people is that they think God reacts the same way they do." And Maria von Trapp, the heroine of *The Sound of Music,* wondered in real life why it happens with some people that a religion of charity gets dwarfed into a religion of chastity.

# The fascination of Jesus

I and many others find two things especially spellbinding about Jesus: (1) his remarkable concern for "people on the edge" and (2) his remarkable insistence that we all need to be forgiven, therefore, we all need to be forgiving.

As a scandalizing "friend of publicans and sinners," Jesus specialized in people who were the social, economic and religious outcasts of his society: sinners in general, prostitutes in particular, lepers (unclean!), unorthodox Samaritans (heretics!), hated tax-collectors, foreign mercenaries and poor widows with no financial power or security.

In a society that downgraded women, he took them very seriously. He idealized "unimportant" people, such as children. He praised the shepherd who leaves the 99 safe sheep and goes looking for the one that is lost. He admired the housewife who wouldn't quit until she found the misplaced coin, the hardly worthwhile coin.

He himself was not easily discouraged. He let himself care about a soldier's servant on the verge of death, about a

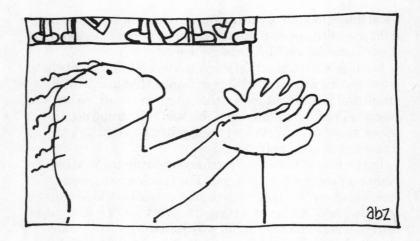

girl who had just expired, about the only son of a widow on his way to burial and about his friend Lazarus, already entombed and decaying.

(And you, my Friend with AIDS: are you not on the edge? — pushed to the edge of your health, of your life expectancy, of your endurance, of your finances, suddenly shoved to the edge of despair, to the edge of the tolerance of your friends, your family, your employer, society . . . and teetering on the cutting edge of expected bouts of illness and perhaps of temptations to suicide.)

How does one explain the astonishing attitude of Jesus toward the marginal people, the down-and-out people, the people who were "despised and rejected" (as the Messiah himself was due to be when he made his appearance)? I think he was warning us that power tends to give powerful people a very dangerous idea of what is genuinely important in life and what makes people genuinely worthwhile.

The same warning goes for healthy people and their health, wealthy people and their wealth, charming people and their charm, popular people and their popularity, successful people and their success, bright people and their brains. In his centerpiece sermon, Jesus declared: "Blessed are those who know that they are poor." Is that because a person will look for genuine wealth once he knows what phony wealth is? And because man's bankrupt despair is God's enriching opportunity?

Jesus put the matter in a few plain words himself: "A person's life does not consist in the abundance of what he possesses." In what, then, does the value of human life consist? It resides inalienably in the built-in dignity with which all human beings are freely endowed by their creator. It is a humbling dignity that needs to be honored by everybody if human affairs are not to go dreadfully wrong. Even when we dislike ourselves intensely, that worth and beauty still persist. It's like a bright shadow that we can't throw off, a golden net from which we cannot leap.

In contrast to the steel-hearted world and its what's-in-it-for-me standards, Jesus saw God's love for human beings as "unconditional" — it doesn't depend on our being worthy of it or even on our behaving worthily of it. By the same token, human beings are most Godlike and Christ-like when their love for another and their service to another are also "unconditional" — that is, when that love and service don't narrowly depend on what the giver is going to get out of the giving. (I'm thinking of Father Damien and his lepers, Mother Teresa, Brother Francis of Assisi and such.)

It is, rather, a love based on the divine beauty indelibly stamped on every human existence. Wrote Alan Watts, "The thing is to see in all faces the masks of God."

(In your face, dear Friend, I would try to see God wounded and in many ways defenseless, wondering whether He can be loved for Himself and not for some lesser reason. As Mother Teresa says, an AIDS patient is Christ Himself in distressing disguise.)

The second main astonishment about Jesus was his interest in mercy and forgiveness. When he preached the beatitudes in his sermon on the mount, he proclaimed, "Blessed are the merciful, for they shall obtain mercy." At the heart of the prayer he composed for his followers, he enshrined the words: "Forgive us our trespasses as we forgive those who trespass against us." He warned, "Judge not, that you may not be judged," and, "With what measure you measure, it shall be measured unto you."

He also warned that we would be in major trouble unless we learned to forgive one another from the heart. On the other hand, he promised, "If you forgive others the wrongs they have done to you, your Father in heaven will also forgive you." That may well be history's most priceless promise.

When his disciple Peter thought he was being generous by suggesting that he would be willing to forgive somebody seven times, Jesus said the recommended number was seventy times seven times. (That's 490.) In what is my all-time favorite gospel story, Jesus stares at the self-righteous people who want to kill an adulterous woman and ingeniously suggests, "Let him who is without sin cast the first stone."

Charles Dickens thought the parable of the prodigal son was the most admirable story in all literature. As you may recall, its twenty verses are about a father who lets his son be free enough to make a mess of his life, but who then takes his "prodigal" (wasteful) son back into his home again without even letting the young man finish his words of apology — his "Act of Contrition" as we Catholics would say.

And when Jesus himself was being nailed to the cross, he practiced what he preached by praying for his executioners, "Father, forgive them; for they know not what they do."

In my general experience, there are initially only two kinds of people: those who sin and those who are not truly tempted. Many are spared certain temptations because some aspects of their human nature (such as righteous wrath and a healthy sensuality) are frozen and have never thawed enough to be either blessings or problems. So in many cases "We atone for the sins that we're most inclined to, by condemning the ones that we have no mind to."

## A two-way street

What was the meaning of this obsession of Jesus with mercy and forgiveness? I think Jesus regarded the holiness and purity and majesty of God as so awesome and absolute — have you ever gazed into the Grand Canyon? — that each one of us is bound to fall colossally short when it comes to dealing appropriately with God and with His mysterious presence in our world, in our neighbor, and in our own hearts and minds and consciences. As St. Paul phrased it: "We have all fallen short of the glory of God." (In fact, we really can't help it.)

Hence we all desperately need the mercy of God, which (thank God!) He is eager to lavish on us. ("God will forgive me — that's His business," wrote the poet Heinrich Heine.) In the light of the millions of dollars in existential debt that God so readily forgives us, we lose the right to be stingy about the pennies in pardon we owe one another.

A wonderful old priest who was for many years the chaplain at Baltimore's Mercy Hospital was famous for the tenderness with which he heard the confessions of patients. There was even a joke that if you confessed you had murdered your sweet and ancient mother, he would argue in your defense, "But surely, my son, you were most grievously provoked!"

I've made these remarks about Jesus and his view of God, not because I presume you share them or must share them, but simply because countless human beings in their moments of crisis have been uniquely nourished by these visions of human dignity and divine pity. Also, his words about mercy can inspire compassion for people with AIDS.

## Feeling guilty

The ideas of mercy and forgiveness naturally imply the uniquely human experience of guilt. I wish to make one vital point very clear: When in this letter I refer to forgiveness, I am not saying you should feel guilty because you have AIDS, because you may be gay or a drug-user, or because you may have had gay or extramarital experiences, either selectively or randomly. It is neither my intention nor my right to dictate to someone else's conscience. In any case, I must distinguish between objective standards and a person's subjective responsibility. (People's characters do grow faster, though, if they have excuses but refuse to use them.)

In these pages I am referring to the guilt of Everyman — our individual and collective guilt for moral and spiritual failures, for lack of concern and human empathy. To repeat St. Paul, "We have *all* fallen short." A non-Catholic once told me he would like to go to confession — not for any particular sin, "but for my whole damned life." Many of us have such moments, and we need to believe that cleansing and fresh starts are possible.

The philosopher and atheist Jean Paul Sartre believed that the history of every person is the story of a failure. "We are made in no fit proportion to the universal occasion," as the poet Christopher Fry put it.

No doubt, we suffer from neurotic guilts and irrational guilts and guilts sometimes caused by debatable norms of culture or of a given society. But I (and most people) believe there is such a thing as authentic guilt.

I don't think this would be a better planet if all such guilt were repressed. The guards and doctors at Nazi concentration camps would have been much better off (as would, for instance, their tens of thousands of gay victims) had they suffered more pangs of authentic guilt.

It is no secret that sex is a uniquely productive source of guilt — both neurotic and (I would say) authentic. Sex is a powerful energy with powerful consequences, some creative, some destructive. In our quest for pleasure, for intimacy, for a loving relationship that will soften our loneliness and help fill up our emptiness, many of us find only too many opportunities to turn sex into something selfish, manipulative, harmful and eventually self-defeating.

**10**

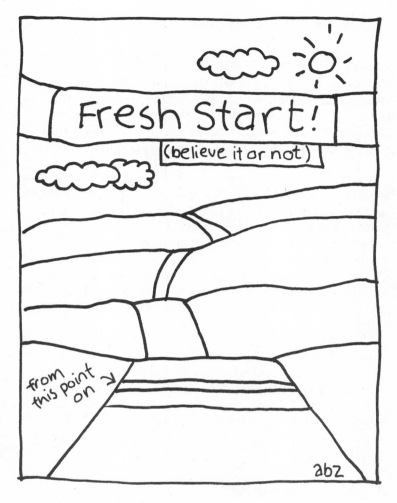

This is true of all sex, whether straight or gay. The mercy Jesus preached pertains to authentic sexual guilt and all other authentic guilts. It aims to heal as well the wounds inflicted by neurotic guilt. In any case, the ideas of Jesus are heart-stretching and breathtaking. The poet Annie Dillard recommends that when you read the Gospels you wear a seatbelt and a helmet because the words of Jesus can hit you like a whirlwind.

# After the first shock

I think I can safely presume that when you were diagnosed as having AIDS, you and your whole world were shaken to the roots. I'm fairly sure such would be my reaction as well. I don't have the gall to presume to tell you how you should react now that the first shock has passed. But I'd like to say something about how I hope I would react, about the ideas I hope I'd try to keep in my rattled head.

The poet W.H. Auden once said, "Life is a blessing, even when you cannot bless it." I know a blind psychiatrist who astonishes with a similar claim: "Blindness is a gift, but you have to know how to unwrap it."

French novelist Leon Bloy acutely observed that "a world without suffering is a world without revelation." Conversely, to a person suffering from a sickness such as AIDS, certain things will be revealed: who his true friends are, or who at least are the bravest and tenderest among them.

Unveiled, too, along with rejections, will be the capacity of some family members and even of strangers to show unquestioning acceptance and energetic compassion. Remember what Blanche Du Bois says in *A Streetcar Named Desire*: "I have always depended on the kindness of strangers." Even as you suffer the pain of some rebuffs, be prepared to be surprised by the goodness of the most unlikely people.

# A gift for others

As an AIDS patient, I would try to make myself realize I was potentially an occasion of amazing grace and even of heroism for some people — especially family members and friends and nurses and doctors and counselors and chaplains and volunteers. I hope I'd graciously let them love me and be good to me. For their own sweet sakes.

When a person has clearly been an instrument of grace,

the Quakers like to say, "Friend, thou hast been used." An acquaintance of mine — whom I thought was quite a worldling — once surprised me by saying with admiration that being religious means being willing to be used. (Conversely, "useless to God" was a phrase which terrified the poet George Herbert.)

Christianity offers a unique and awesome mystique of suffering according to which each of us is summoned to carry on the saving work of Christ. Thus St. Paul could write, "In my flesh I am taking my turn in filling up what is lacking in the tribulations of Christ." He could thus lovingly assert, "I rejoice in my sufferings for you."

Such is the relevance of Good Friday, for "we are all contemporaries of that immortal day," and each of us is nailed to the cross of being who we are. Through us, Christ hangs on the cross till the end of time. (Said a boy who was mesmerized by a large, realistic church crucifix, "He's still bleeding!") Thus, all this human suffering is redemptive, especially when it is undeserved.

The same hard-pressed Leon Bloy wrote that "there are places in the heart which do not yet exist. Suffering must enter in before these places can come to be." (I wonder whether the movie *Places in the Heart* took its title from that remark.) This creativity of suffering applies not only to the one who suffers, but also to those who seek to lessen the suffering by sharing it.

The heart-melting and throat-lumping book, *Goodbye, I Love You*, by Carol Lynn Pearson, tells of a woman who took back her gay husband when he was dying of AIDS. (Talk about unconditional-love-made-flesh!) She herself was mightily touched to discover that even very strict fellow Mormons could open their hearts to a situation they might have been expected to deem sinful and shameful: "People who won't even drink coffee have a hard time understanding homosexuality and AIDS, but they don't have a hard time understanding suffering and need."

Another woman who suffered a devastating loss later confided, "Since God cannot fill the soul until it is emptied

**13**

of all trivial concerns, a great grief is a tremendous bonfire in which all the trash of life is consumed." I heard a former drug addict, a young woman scarcely in her 30s, gratefully declare that AIDS had throttled her awake to the genuine meaning of life for the first time in her life. ("In a dark time," wrote the troubled poet Theodore Roethke, "the eye begins to see." For sure: You can't see the myriad stars or their hypnotic patterns in the noonday glare of that one minor star called the sun.)

Her illness has cured this woman spiritually from being a vacuum cleaner for herself into being a heatlamp for shivering others. Especially through her new work with drug abusers and other AIDS patients, she has gained a sense of focus and of function that she never knew before and that she might have died at a ripe old age without ever knowing.

"Most people," it has been lamented, "die with their music still in them." If I came down with AIDS, I hope I'd work hard to get as much of my music out as I could. (Is it true that what we fear is not so much dying as never having really lived?)

## Dancing on the edge

It's an old story that a crisis can bring out the saving best in people. (A boy remains a boy until there's need for a man.) The Chinese word for "crisis" is (I'm told) composed of the signs for "danger" and "opportunity." The essence of the human spirit is "its ability to dance on the edge of a crisis."

Dr. Shervert H. Frazier, who directs the National Institute of Mental Health, has noted that some AIDS patients "cope uncommonly well" with their disease, "drawing on wellsprings of strength that nourish other patients and the staff as well." Margaret Staudacher, a nurse in a San Francisco AIDS ward, said of her patients, "It's amazing how they handle it. Sometimes they give me

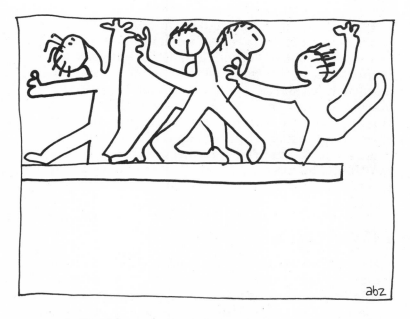

strength. It's the most rewarding nursing I've done in 30 years."

Perhaps these patients have always understood that the task of human existence is not to have a winning hand, but to play well the hand you've been handed. (I realize that one of the things we've been handed is the capacity to deal ourselves a raw deal, accidentally or recklessly or even deliberately.) I have a doctor friend who says that when he finally gets an appointment with God he plans to say, "Well, I played the cards you dealt me. And I tried not to complain."

What of my grief at the prospect of dying young — or at least younger than I wanted to? I hope I'd consider the fact that the longest life is short, and the shortest life is miraculous. None of us can do anything certain about extending the length of our lives, but we do have some control over how deep and wide and high they get to be. (Three out of four isn't bad.)

Although sorry to leave so soon this inexhaustibly

**15**

fascinating planet — but wouldn't anytime be too soon? —
I'd try to think of the countless human beings throughout
history who lived a shorter life than mine has already
been: fetuses in the womb, babes in infancy, teenagers in
bloody battles and senseless car accidents and drug
overdoses. In how many eras of war and plague and
starvation has the average person lived a life far more
"solitary, poor, nasty, brutish and short" than mine has
been. I hope I wouldn't discover that I've been "spoiled"
into the quaint notion that somehow or other I was entitled
to favors never bestowed on millions of my planetary
siblings.

## Life as fair and unfair

As President Kennedy said, and then went on to demon-
strate: Life is unfair. But what if life is not meant to be fair,
not, at least, according to our rather short-sighted and
self-centered human standards? The poet John Keats, who
died at 25 after a life of generosity to his orphaned siblings
and his friends, believed this world was meant to be a vale
of soul-making.

When, as an AIDS patient, I fell into moods of self-pity
(as I expect I would), I hope I'd be teased by these words:
"To believe in God is to know that all the rules are fair and
that in the end there will be some wonderful surprises."

I don't mean to be too hard on self-pity. It usually has the
advantage of being sincere! At times we might actually
underdo it: "My own heart let me more have pity on,"
priest-poet Gerard Manley Hopkins once advised his
hard-on-self self.

But if I thought AIDS was my own fault? What of the
way I've messed up my life and perhaps the lives of others?
These are megaton thoughts, and with them can come
pulverizing guilt, guilt too destructive for any human
being to bear. Here, the person who believes in God has a
crucial advantage. (To be honest, though, I guess if a
person truly considers all life to be an absurd flash in the

**16**

pan, then lethal infections, pain, early death and suicide wouldn't really make all that much difference anyway — at least in theory.)

There was a sunny 14th-century holy man named Master Eckhart. One of his favorite urgings was this: "Let God be God." His point was that, in so many ways that we can't even help, that we never asked for, we are weak, deaf, mute, blind, sinful, fallible, pitiful creatures. (Who can fathom the extent to which chemistry, biology, heredity, environment and "the unconscious" influence the good choices we think we freely make, and the bad choices we think those evil-doers cold-heartedly make?)

Our task, therefore, is clearly not to play God, not to try to puzzle out the big picture (much less orchestrate it), not to "unscrew" the inscrutable, not to turn all evils to good, not to undo personally all our sins and stupidities, not to assume that the future cannot redeem the past, not to have figured out and cared about, ahead of time, all the splintered consequences of our complexly motivated actions.

No. Let God be God — especially after the fact, and after we have done our reasonable best to repair and head off any damages. It's God's job to manage the billions of multicolored threads comprising the gigantic tapestry of human history.

As for my own small patch of tapestry, I usually see only the underside, and I see it up much too close. You'd be closer to the words, but not to their meaning, if your eyes were pressed against this page. You probably know the proverb that God can write straight with crooked lines. But even divine penmanship needs perspective. And don't judge a mystery writer until you've read his last lines.

Our role is essentially to be as loving and honest and forgiving toward one another as we can be "in the corner where we are," in the brief time that even the longest-lived of us will tarry on this terrain. "What does the Lord require of thee?" asks the prophet Micah. "To do the right, to love mercy and to walk humbly with your God."

"Let God be God": That's the mantra I'd plan to recite to

**17**

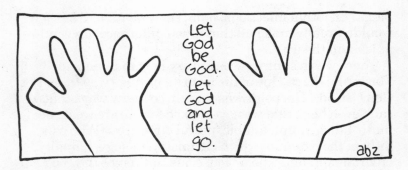

myself, hoping at last to get the very large point. A similar mantra would be: "Let God and let go." St. Paul was enough of a cosmic optimist to insist that all things — including AIDS — work together unto good for those who love God. In that category, I would unquestioningly include all those people who love goodness and prize it, even if they don't always practice it. So let God do the king-size worrying, and let us let go of our tiny and largely fruitless frettings.

## All will be well

Another holy person of the 14th century, Julian of Norwich, picked up where Master Eckhart left off. She summarized her mystical revelations by promising: "Sin is behovely (of use), but all shall be well, and all shall be well, and all manner of thing shall be well." In the meantime, in the midst of a harsh existence, she had discovered life, love and light as God's essence: "In life is marvelous homeliness; in love: gentle courtesy; in light: infinite, endless kindness." In her spirit, a friend of mine likes to prophesy: "No good thing will be lost; no dear thing will be forgotten; every human thing will connect."

Maybe at this moment you find it hard — or impossible — to believe in a personal, caring God, or at least to have an overmastering faith in his mercy. ("The Lord loves those who trust in his mercy — the mercy that is the greatest of his works," sings the Psalmist.) But on this score the Gospel itself provides a perfect prayer: "I believe, Lord; help Thou my unbelief!"

A wounded man lost in the woods might not believe there is anyone around to hear him, but he would still most likely cry out. I ardently urge you to try some shouting—if only in the form of a quiet, even wordless prayer sinking down from your own pre-rational, pre-skeptical roots to the Roots of Reality.

A young monk once asked his Zen master to teach him how to pray. The master took him to a river bank, told him to kneel over the water, hold his breath and not resist. Then the master plunged the young man's face into the water and held it there for what seemed an eternity. Finally, he extracted the head of his disciple, who sucked in gaspingly a breath that seemed destined for his toes. "That," explained the old master, "is how you pray!"

## The value of anger

Don't suppose you can't pray to God because of your anger toward him (even if you suspect that at bottom the anger may be irrational). Go ahead, voice your anger and make that anger your prayer. You'll be in first-class company. The giants of the Bible didn't hesitate to complain to God.

In more recent times the plain-speaking St. Teresa of Avila was once becoming very much frustrated in her efforts to do good. When the Lord appeared to her, she complained of his treatment. He said he treated all his friends that way. Back she snapped, "No wonder you have so few!"

As you may know, Dr. Elisabeth Kübler-Ross has made a specialty of dealing with death and dying. I once heard her address a group of nurses. She told them, "Don't try to keep sick or bereaved people from venting their rage at God. He can take it." The audience burst into applause.

Anger is a unique source of energy. As a God-given part

of our natures, wrath is not a sin in itself. The virtue of meekness is not meant to destroy anger, but to keep it from becoming senselessly destructive. Anger-energy helps to knit a person together inside and armors that person with a needed feeling of protection against what appears to be threatening.

St. Thomas Aquinas noted that anger is often the first step in courage. I hope I wouldn't deprive myself of that first step, even if I were later given the gift to develop a more serene, embracing attitude toward my illness.

## Your picture of God

As you go about deciding whether and how you believe in God and trying to determine what relationship he has to you and your illness, try to become aware of the picture you have of him in your mind. Maybe, because of painful associations, it's the picture you're really having trouble with — and ought to! Each of us is free, of course, to picture God as a competitor and a kill-joy, as someone who is out to get us, out to get us to say "Uncle" (instead of "Father") and to zap us if we don't.

But we are equally free to unmask him at the roots of everything true and beautiful and good that we've ever experienced or dreamed of in our lives. We are free to think of him as an enveloping energy that is benign and healing beyond all imagining. When we pray, we invite that energy to invade us ever more penetratingly, and through us to love and heal the wider world.

The difference between adult religion and infantile magic is this: A child (of any age) uses magic to try to get God to do what the child wants; an adult (of any age) uses religion to trying to do what God wants.

And what does God want? The aforementioned Juliana wrote, "Wouldst thou wit thy Lord's meaning? Wit it well. Love is his meaning." For his part, St. John of the Cross taught that "in the evening of life we shall all be judged on love."

purpose of prayer, then, is not to change God. He
ly knows what we need, Jesus assured us. Prayer
es people, and people change things — to the extent
ley can. For the balance, a child's rhyme can serve
: "They are blest who do their best and leave the rest
"

## picture of your illness

ictures in our mind can also be critical when we
our illnesses. When a person has AIDS, it will be
easy for him or her to view that illness and all its
consequences as a heartless, ferocious dragon.
normally do with dragons, of course, is run like
them. I know this is easy for me to say, but I am
certain that a supremely saving wisdom lies
hidden in these three words: Hug your dragon (even while
allowing for a superb surprise).

When we run from a situation and presume we are
totally defenseless against it, we make that dragon more
massive and dreadful than it really is. In the long run, the
fearing and the running can be worse than the dragon
itself. If I could wish a gift upon you, it would be this: that
you may soon discover the strength and serenity that can
come from trying to hug your dragon.

This hugging is what Jesus meant when he said, "Take
up your cross, and follow me." It is what Jesus did in the
garden of Gethsemane when in a bloody sweat he prayed,
"Thy will be done." Hugging your dragon is what the
famous words of the poet Dante suggest: "In his will is our
peace: That is the sea to which all things created run."

Rainer Maria Rilke, a master poet of our own century,
wrote these arresting words: "Those ancient myths about
dragons which at the last minute turn into princesses,
perhaps they are saying something true. Perhaps all the
dragons of our lives are princesses who are only waiting to
see us once beautiful and brave. Perhaps everything

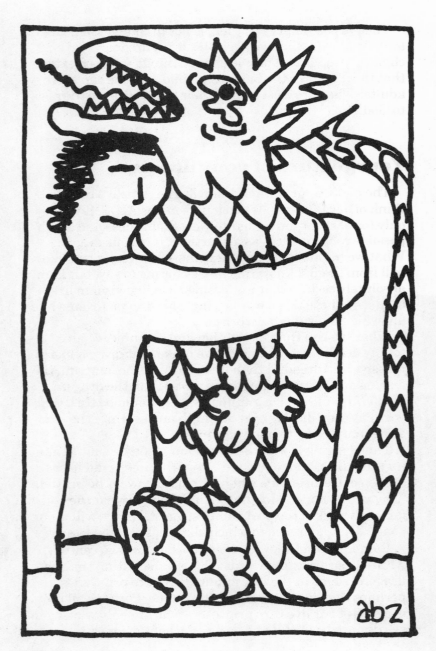

terrible is, in its deepest being, something helpless that needs help from us."

If you feel you cannot hug your dragon right away, let that be your dragon, and hug that present incapacity. The nerve-wracked French novelist Marcel Proust came to this conclusion: "We are healed of a suffering only by experiencing it to the full." This experiencing takes time. "Give time time," the Portuguese say.

Finally, there is the picture you have of yourself as a patient with AIDS. Inside each of us is a sometimes panicky child, and several kinds of adults. You have probably seen in your lifetime a frightened and perhaps injured puppy. Your instinct was to pick it up, to bring it close to the warmth of your breast and to pet it gently and soothingly. Surely, you wouldn't kick it and add to its pains!

Once in my own life, when I was feeling especially fearful and the wrecking balls of self-disappointment were pounding on my nervous system, I was amazed to experience an instant, palpable relief simply by thinking of myself as just such a petrified puppy and then picking myself up and tenderly petting myself. (Curiously, we weaken our dragon by hugging it and strengthen our puppy by petting it.)

Many of us have a fearsome, unforgiving prison guard lurking inside us. (Is he our picture of God?) We also have a miraculously understanding and forgiving parent, strong as a father, tender as a mother. (In the book of the prophet Isaiah, God says, "Even if a mother forget her child, I will never forget you. See, I have written your name on the palm of my hands.") We need to put that composite parent to work more than we do — especially when the little child in us stands bruised and terrified.

I know a medical secretary who signs off all her phone calls with words even more helpful than "Have a nice day." Her prescription: "Be kind to yourself." That is advice a patient with AIDS sorely needs to take, no matter what the cause or consequences of his or her illness.

Were I such a patient — after I had been kind enough to afford myself time to work through my shock and fear and rage and whatever self-lacerations — I hope I'd be ready to welcome the really Olympic-class gift: the willingness to forgive those who have injured me, failed me, condemned me, rejected me, fled from me. As has been mentioned, such failures are still pennies in the spiritual economics of Jesus, mere fractions in his mathematics of mercy.

## AIDS of the spirit

There is an AIDS of the body, but there is also an AIDS of the spirit that can afflict seemingly "healthy" human beings. In their reaction to AIDS patients, people (especially those who profess to be religious and decent) should be immune to hatred and contempt and vengeance and rash judgment and cruelty and cowardice.

In their first reaction to a shock of revelation, however, people should be permitted to say something mean that they probably don't really mean. Thus, when a 22-year-old son told his mother simultaneously that he was gay and had AIDS, she said she had perpetrated just one mammoth mistake in her life: not having had an abortion 23 years earlier. People in shock are not always at their noblest.

But sometimes their immune systems fail altogether, and almost against their wills they fall victim to a deadly virus of the spirit. But their virus is curable, and the rejected person's willingness to forgive in the spirit of Jesus may well be a decisive part of the cure — and of his or her own heart-cure as well.

There's a companion gift to this forgiveness of others. Emotionally, it is probably part of a package deal. Anne Morrow Lindbergh, a woman acquainted with sorrow, was once visiting the bedside of Edward Sheldon, a promising playwright who was striken in midlife with paralyzing arthritis and blindness. She told him she thought the ideal critical attitude would be "black and white about oneself, but gray about the rest of the world."

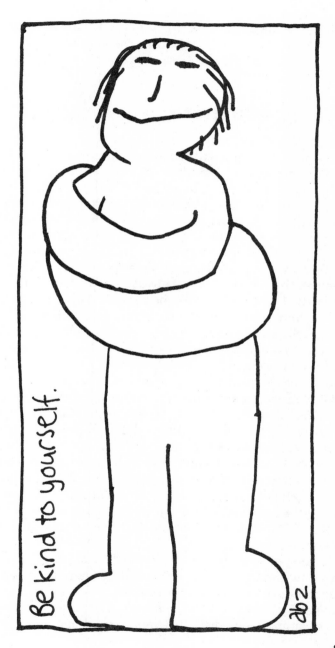

Be kind to yourself.

"Oh, no," he quickly corrected her. "You must be gray about yourself, too. You must forgive yourself too. That is the hardest thing of all."

## Coping with the future

As an AIDS patient, I hope I would leave my past to God's mercy, my present to his love and my future to his providence. I hope I would live in day-tight or even hour-tight compartments, refusing to dwell on the trials that might lie ahead. Although not always true, there's a point to the saying: "Life is hard by the yard, but a cinch by the inch." By contrast, those who cross their bridges before they come to them have to pay the toll twice — at least.

Here are two parables that have rescued me when I've dreaded the future. You are about to drive over a long, rocky road. You think of all the rocks and stones that lie ahead, and in your mind you combine all of them into a giant blockade. You are overwhelmed in your imagination because you doubt your car can handle "all those obstacles." But the emboldening truth is that, in reality, you will encounter them only one by one. Divide and conquer.

Or, you are driving down a pitch-dark country road. You imagine "all that darkness" engulfing you and facing you. Once again you feel overwhelmed. But as you approach each small section of the road, you will bring your headlights with you. In all that paralyzing darkness, the only illumination you truly need is just enough for the manageable patch of road immediately ahead of you. Keep your battery in good shape and you will have the vision you need. What is crucial is not the darkness without but the brightness within.

In the Lord's Prayer it's "our daily bread" that is asked for — not next week's or next month's. There is no deep-freeze for grace. It is always and only fresh. In their 40-year journey through the desert, the chosen people were commanded normally to gather just enough manna

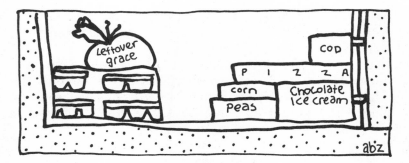

for the day ahead. And that was enough for their needs. Enough is enough!

Instead of stockpiling thoughts of the possible trials ahead, I hope I would try to reinforce my spirits with thoughts of all the unpurchasable gifts with which life had already surprised and enriched me, with memories, too, of the needed people who had shown up in my life at the most blessedly unexpected times. Oprah Winfrey likes to say that God may seem maddeningly slow, but he is never late. If that's truly so, it may be partly so because, as a poet discovered, "good grows wild and wide, has shades, is nowhere none." And wears many human masks.

Granted, there is a mystery of evil in the world. But there is also a mystery of good. Evil is not the only word. There are compelling reasons for believing it is not the final word. And how often we discover that it is not even the right word!

Is there any human being who has not suffered a setback that turned out to be one of the most productive gifts of his or her life? Mary Fraser, head nurse in a West Coast AIDS ward, made this discovery: "Some really blossom here. They start making amends with their families and friends. I had one guy tell me his AIDS was the best thing that ever happened to him."

Unquestionably, the darkest evil can become the creative foil for the brightest goodness and courage. When the great plague struck England in the 1660s, there was an outbreak of it in the little village of Eyam. People were going to flee the town. But their 28-year-old Anglican rector spoke up, pointing out that those who fled might well be taking the plague with them.

The heroic pastor persuaded his heroic parishioners to quarantine themselves in order to spare others. Of the 350 villagers, 259 (including the pastor's wife) died before the plague had spent itself. A recent service in honor of those townspeople noted that they "counted not their lives dear to themselves, but laid them down for their friends" — friends they didn't even know!

In our own century, a family of Christians in the Polish town of Nowy Korczyn hid a total of nine Jews for 900 days beneath the floorboards of a storage room in their home. During all that time, in a trench the size of two coffins, these stowaways never stood up, never saw the light of day, never spoke above a whisper. If one wanted to turn his body, everyone had to turn.

Who could ever have anticipated the enduring courage of the hiders or the courageous endurance of the hidden? In a time of unspeakable terror, these were nine who survived — though they understandably begged at times for their protectors to give them poisoned bread or guns for self-destruction.

You, my Friend with AIDS, have probably thought about suicide, or may do so later. A seminary teacher of mine used to say, "A man must be pretty hard-pressed to take his own life." Who should dare to sit in judgment on any hard-pressed person? But if and when you suffer the temptation to decide how long your life will be (and, therefore, how fruitful it can be), I pray that you will take into account the kinds of thoughts these pages offer and recall the role of the unexpected in human existence.

In the face of such a temptation, I hope I would remember the words of the heroic Russian poet Osip Mandelstam, who died in one of Stalin's prisons: "You must live out your whole life in order to realize that it doesn't belong to you."

When the genius Buckminster Fuller was on the verge

of self-destruction in 1927, a voice within him successfully protested in amazingly similar words: "You do not have the right to eliminate yourself. You do not belong to you. You belong to the universe."

## Dying: the last stage of growing

Rounding out one's life in this visible universe can be a giant step in the process of becoming fully human. Every stage of human growth involves the giving up of security and comfort for a better sort of freedom that usually comes at a cost. Giving up is hard, and that's why growing up is hard. "There are so many little dyings that it doesn't matter which of them is death," wrote Kenneth Patchen.

The law of losing in order to gain applies to the fetus when it is forced to leave the snug safety of the womb; to the crawling babe who first begins to walk; to the homebound, protected child who faces a classroom of competing strangers; to the teenager who risks asking for a date, leaving home for college or joining the army; to the single person who takes on the commitments of marriage and parenthood; to the aging or ailing person who approaches "the valley of the shadow of death." (There would, by the way, be no valleys without mountains, no shadows without light, no death without life.)

## Who holds the future

Religious people do not know what the future holds, but they lodge their faith in one who holds the future. Graham Greene once said a saint is like someone who enters a theater just at the happy ending of a terrifying movie. Then she sees it from the start, like the rest of the audience, who didn't come early. The saint is just as confused as anybody else as to how all the parts fit together and how evil will be overcome, but she knows the happy secret. Faith can give even the non-saint a sense of that secret.

It has been pointed out that, in the Bible, God did not actually tell the patriarch Abraham to leave the known and, safe and to "go" into the unknown and the dangerous. Rather, because God himself promised to show Abraham a new land, he was inviting him to "come" into the future. God is a freer tomorrow coaxing us this privileged today out of an imprisoning yesterday.

Think of the father who holds his child by its hands and lets it stand on his feet as the child stumbles shakily forward and the father walks steadily backward. Or recall an image suggested by the French writer Charles Peguy: A mother teaches her daughter to swim by alternately holding her up in the water and then creatively letting go of her for awhile. Only thus will the parent's power go permanently from outside the child to inside it.

Philosopher John Macmurray makes this distinction between unreal and real religion: "One says, 'Fear not. Trust in God and he will see that none of the things you fear will happen to you.' The other says, 'Fear not. The things you are afraid of may very well happen to you, but they are nothing to be afraid of.'"

The Trappist monk Thomas Merton offered kindred, adaptable advice: "Anxiety is inevitable in an age of crisis like ours. Don't make it worse by deceiving yourself and acting as if you were immune to all inner trepidation. God does not ask you not to feel anxious — but to trust him no matter how you feel."

Wise and holy human beings have always insisted that the goal of our existence is not a long and struggle-free life, but a good and gutsy one. Such a life doesn't require much time, only much love and a measure of timely courage. Of Mary Magdalene, who braved the finger-pointing, nose-lifting, tongue-wagging crowd, Jesus said that she had been forgiven much, because she loved much.

Jesus also said that the tears of the penitent Magdalene had anointed him for death. But no matter how isolated we may feel, we are all of us together in the departure lounge. Granted, Friend, you are having a special kind of near-death experience. Nearly eight million Americans claim to have had near-death experiences in a technical sense.

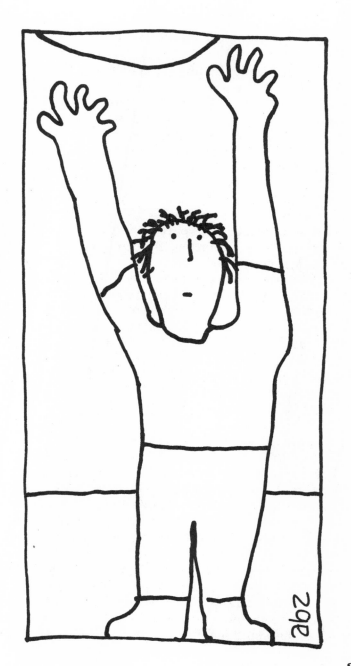

They speak intriguing words of comfort:

> "One definite finding of the research done on these claimants is their diminishing fear of death. Death is experienced as less painful and more peaceful than it is generally conceived to be. Many say they enter a tunnel of darkness and move toward a brilliant white light that emits warmth and love, that they are flooded with knowledge beyond their ordinary capacities, that they discern the pattern or meaning of life: 'I was part of everything in the universe. Everything fit together and made sense to me.'
>
> "Near-death experiences are also a catalyst for spiritual development: The individuals seem to become more self-confident, less materialistic and more giving of themselves." (*New York Times,* Oct. 28, 1986). A century earlier Walt Whitman had guessed, "To die is different from what anyone supposed, and luckier."

## Private gifts

I began writing this letter while staying at the beach in Ocean City, Md. One night the moon rose full over the glittering, wind-wimpled waters. As I gazed out my window, the moon was casting over the sea a golden carpet that appeared to be aimed exactly and exclusively at my balcony.

I imagined a newcomer to the ocean who would see this private wonder and go running up and down the sand inviting other beachdwellers to come to his balcony and savor this unique miracle. If only he took another look at the ocean, he would see that our generous, wily Sister

Moon sends her customized splendor to every locale on the coast.

In these pages, I have tried to share with you the bolts of light that over a period of nearly six decades have come streaming to me as gifts from life itself, from life rafts disguised as books, and from living, loving voices of hard-won wisdom. I hope the sharing has comforted and befriended you to some degree. May these spindrift pages do so again if you honor them with a second reading. (Some ideas are night-blooming flowers with their own mysterious timing).

But — even better — may you keep doing your own looking and listening and pondering and praying (if you can) and discover thereby in the darkness those pathways of energizing light that are lovingly sent to especially you and are stretching to reach you wherever you are.

AIDS is not the only malady that flesh is heir to, and one illness can be healed by another. All bodily life is sooner or later fatal, and the scaffold of our bones does well to wear itself out in the forging of spirit. Still, for most of us it takes courage to live out a destiny that includes the death of the body, even if we believe that such a death is not the last word.

Tennessee Williams wrote about that kind of fortitude in his *Night of the Iguana*:

> How calmly does the orange branch
> Observe the sky begin to blanch:
> Without a cry, without a prayer,
> With no betrayal of despair . . .
>
> O Courage, could you not as well
> Select a second place to dwell —
> Not only in that golden tree
> But in the frightened heart of me?

Unlike that unconscious golden tree, however, many

human beings have found that they can be even more courageous "with a cry and with a prayer" — though they still resist the "carrion comfort," "the rotten luxury" of despair.

Dag Hammarskjöld, once Secretary General of the U.N., gave himself a kindly permission: "Cry. Cry if you must. But do not complain. The path has chosen you. And in the end you will say, Thank you."

That's my prayer and hope for you, embattled Friend: that in the months and years ahead you too will discover your own transfiguring reasons for saying Thank You. I have my reasons for saying, "God bless you," for I am, respectfully,

*Your brother, Joe*

# Other voices

General George Washington had learned the inmost secret of the brave, who train themselves to contemplate in mind the worst that can happen, and resign themselves to it in thought — but never in action.

George Otto Trevelyan

* * *

Though the physicality of death destroys the individual, the idea of death can save him. Contemplate death if you would learn how to live. Kept in mind, death passes into a state of gratitude, of appreciation for the countless givens of existence.

E.M. Forster

* * *

The tragedy of life is not how much we suffer, but how much we miss.

Thomas Carlyle

* * *

Given to my youth, my faith, my sword,
Choice of my heart's desire:
A short life in the saddle, Lord,
Not long life by the fire.

Louise Imogen Guiney

* * *

## Prayer of St. Francis of Assisi

Lord, make me an instrument of thy peace.
Where there is hatred, let me plant love;
where there is injury, pardon;
where there is doubt, faith;
where there is despair, hope;
where there is sadness, joy.

O Divine Master:
grant that I may not so much seek to be consoled
as to console;
to be understood as to understand;
to be loved as to love.

For it is in giving that we receive;
it is in pardoning that we are pardoned;
and it is in dying that we are born to eternal life.

\* \* \*

The Christmas before he died of AIDS, Gerald sat on the couch with his arms around two of the children. When his wife Carol had finished reading *The Other Wise Man*, he spoke:

"I have something for our Christmas program too. I want to lead you in a meditation for peace. Close your eyes, everybody. Feel the energy that is in you, giving you life. Now feel and visualize that energy rising out of you and joining with the energy of all of us together in this room.

"It is a great, glowing mass of energy, of spirit, and rises further now and joins with the energy of everybody everywhere who is doing positive things.

"Now all that energy rises and is joined by the brightest, the most powerful energy of all, that of Christ, and as our light and energy join with his, there is a force that is shining and powerful.

"Now I want you to visualize this great and powerful force moving across the entire world. Wherever it meets war, wherever it meets hate, wherever it meets prejudice, it moves through and dissolves it and leave only peace and love. See it move everywhere: across the entire planet there is at last truly peace on earth."

Carol Lynn Pearson in *Goodbye, I Love You*

* * *

I said to the man who stood at the gate of the year: "Give me a light, that I may tread safely into the unknown."
And he replied: "Go out into the darkness and put your hand into the hand of God. That shall be to you better than light and safer than a known way."

M. Louise Haskins

* * *

We are all falling. This hand's falling too —
all have this falling sickness, none withstands.
And yet there's always One whose gentle hands
this universal falling can't fall through.

Rainer Maria Rilke

* * *

And the disciples of Jesus asked him: "Rabbi, who has sinned, this man or his parents, that he should be born blind?"
Jesus answered: "Neither has this man sinned, nor his parents, but the works of God were to be made manifest in him."

*John: 9:2-4*

* * *

I don't believe in miracles. But I rely on them.

Words of the old Jewish grandfather in the<br>Canadian film, *Songs My Father Never Taught Me*

* * *

**37**

Do no seek death. Death will find you. But seek the
road which makes death a fulfillment.

Dag Hammarskjöld

\* \* \*

Any day is a good day to be born on, a good day to die
on.

Pope John XXIII at 80

\* \* \*

Undying Father, boundless Ocean of Being: You are
the God Who was, the God Who is, the God Who is to
come. Teach me to leave the past to Your mercy, the
present to Your love, the future to Your providence. Let
me not look back in anger, nor forward in fear, but coax
me gently to look around in constant, grateful aware-
ness.

\* \* \*

About midnight Paul and Silas were praying and
singing hymns to God, and the other prisoners were
listening to them. Suddenly there was a violent
earthquake, which shook the prison to its foundations.
At once all the doors opened, and the chains fell off all
the prisoners.
    The jailer woke up, and when he saw the prison
doors open, he thought the prisoners had escaped. So
he pulled out his sword and was about to kill himself.
But Paul shouted at the top of his voice *Do not harm
yourself: we are all here!*

*Acts 16:25-28*

\* \* \*

In the icy hurricane, in the tempest of collapse, all
the doors spring open, the foundations of our prison are

shaken, and from the profoundest darkness of the world, from our bitterness and our deepest darkness a cry of help comes to the helpless: a voice is heard — the voice that binds all that has been to all that is to come, the voice that binds our loneliness to all other loneliness. It is not the voice of dread and doom; it falters in the silence of the Eternal Word and yet is borne on by it, raised high over the clamour of the non-existent. It is the voice of man and of the tribes of men, the voice of comfort and hope and immediate love: "Do thyself no harm! for we are all here."

Hermann Broch in *The Sleepwalkers*

\* \* \*

The Lord is my shepherd; I have everything I need.
He lets me rest where the fields are green,
lets me quench my thirst
in the freshness of quiet streams.
Thus He renews my vigor,
thus He guides me in paths that are sure.
Even though I pass through the valley of death's
    own shadow,
I will not fear, good Lord,
for there You are, beside me,
with Your shepherd's staff for my stout defense.
You make a feast of food for me,
while those who would starve me watch.
You welcome me as an honored guest
and fill to the brim my cravings.
I know that Your loving kindness
will shepherd me securely down all my days,
that where You dwell will always be home to me.

*Psalm 23 (22)*

\* \* \*

MOSCOW (AP): February 8, 1987: Irena Ratushinskaya, a 32-year-old dissident poet, was released from a Russian prison after three and a half years. During most of that time she was denied any writing materials. So with burnt match sticks she carved 250 new poems on bars of soap. "I would read it and read it until it was committed to memory, then with one washing of my hands, it would be gone."

\* \* \*

Even in our sleep, pain that cannot forget
falls drop by drop upon the heart;
until, in our despair and against our will,
comes wisdom by the awful grace of God.

> Aeschylus: carved at the
> grave of Robert F. Kennedy

\* \* \*

In the middle of winter I learned at last that I carried within myself an invincible summer.

> Albert Camus

\* \* \*

I asked God for strength, that I might achieve;
I was made weak, that good might be achieved in me. . .

I asked for health, that I might do greater things;
I was given infirmity, that I might do better things. . .

I asked for riches, that I might be happy;
I was given poverty, that I might be wise. . .

I asked for power, that I might have praise;
I was given weakness, that I might learn patience. . .

I asked for all things, that I might enjoy life;
I was given life, that I might enjoy all things. . .

I got nothing that I asked for — but everything I had
  hoped for. . .
Almost despite myself, my unspoken prayers were
  answered.

The Lord Himself is in our darkness; all is Light
before Him. The night of pain and fear fades away in
His presence. Seek His Face, and trust always in His
love.

* * *


What they were saying to each other was only: Love
me, love me in spite of all! Whether or not I love you,
whether I am fit to love, whether you are able to love,
even if there is no such thing as love, love me!

Katherine Anne Porter in *Ship of Fools*

* * *


Go to the gods, Alexander. May the River of Ordeal
be as mild as milk to you, and bathe you in light, not
fire. May your dead forgive you. . . You were never
without love; and where you go, may you find it
waiting.

Mary Renault in *The Persian Boy*

* * *


A law of courage to clip and save: The fearless breast
cannot be brave.

* * *


The trouble with most of the world's opinions is that
they are held by people who have never relly been in
trouble.

* * *

A man does not fight merely to win.

> Cyrano de Bergerac in Edmond Rostand's play

\* \* \*

A quiet mind cannot be perplexed or frightened, but goes on in fortune or misfortune, at its own private pace, like a clock in a thunderstorm.

> Robert Louis Stevenson

\* \* \*

Pain and suffering, they are a secret. Kindness and love, they are a secret. But I have found that kindness and love can pay for pain and suffering.

> Alan Paton in *Cry, the Beloved Country*

\* \* \*

Man creates out of his moral wounds.

> Joost A.M. Meerloo

\* \* \*

To live is to suffer. To survive is to find meaning in the suffering.

> Viktor Frankl

\* \* \*

Thou recallest me, and I take my departure while thanking Thee without reserve for having admitted me to this great spectacle of the world.

> Epictetus, the slave philosopher

\* \* \*

It tickleth me about my heart's root that I have seen the world as in my time.

Geoffrey Chaucer's *Wife of Bath*

\* \* \*

I was luckily on hand for the sole performance of today.

Steve Herrick

\* \* \*

We have so little time to be born to this moment.

St. John Perse

\* \* \*

"I taught you to love your brother."
"There ain't nothing left to love."
"There's always something left to love. And if you ain't learned that, you ain't learned nothin'."

Lorraine Hansberry in *A Raisin in the Sun*

\* \* \*

This is the simple truth: that to live is to find oneself lost. He who accepts that has already begun to find himself, to be on firm ground.

Ortega y Gasset

\* \* \*

They shall not grow old as we that are left grow old;
Age shall not weary them, nor the years condemn.

War Memorial Inscription:
All Hallows Church, London

\* \* \*

Invited or not, God is present.

Inscription over Carl Jung's doorway

* * *

You feel you are hedged in. You dream of escape. But beware of mirages. . . If you run away from yourself, your prison will run with you and press even closer from the wind of your flight. But if you go down deep into yourself, the prison will disappear.

Gustave Thibon

* * *

In entering into the abyss himself, a man may show as reckless a courage as those who died on the field of battle.

William Butler Yeats

* * *

Courage is fear that has said its prayers.

* * *

When God erases, He is beginning to write.

Jacques Benigne Bossuet

* * *

Only the hand that erases can write the true thing.

Master Eckhart

* * *

Wisdom keeps you from making mistakes, and comes from having made lots of them.

Bernard Baruch

* * *

**44**

Pain makes man think.
Thought makes man wise.
Wisdom makes life endurable.

Sakini in John Patrick's *Teahouse of the August Moon*

\* \* \*

### The Lord's Prayer

Our Father, Who art in heaven,
hallowed be Thy name.
Thy kingdom come;
Thy will be done on earth as it is in heaven.
Give us this day our daily bread,
And forgive us our trespasses as we forgive
    those who trespass against us.
And lead us not into temptation, but deliver us
    from evil.
(For thine is the kingdom, and the power, and
    the glory, forever.)

*Matthew 6:9-11*

\* \* \*

The chain of evil can be broken only by one who is
willing to sacrifice himself in Christlike fashion, to
absorb evil and suffering into himself, without yielding
to the temptation of causing others to suffer.

Simone Weil

\* \* \*

I rejoice in my sufferings for you, and in my flesh I
am taking my turn in filling up what is lacking in the
tribulations of Christ.

St. Paul (Colossians 1:24)

\* \* \*

**45**

There was a man who had two sons. The younger one said to him: "Father, give me my share of the property now." So the man divided his property between his two sons.

After a few days the younger son sold his part of the property and left home with the money. He went to a country far away, where he wasted his money in reckless living. He spent everything he had.

Then a severe famine spread over that country, and he was left without a thing. So he went to work for one of the citizens of that country, who sent him out to his farm to take care of the pigs. He wished he could fill himself with the bean pods the pigs ate, but no one gave him anything to eat.

At last he came to his senses and said: "All my father's workers have more than they can eat, and here I am about to starve! I will get up and go to my father and say: "Father I have sinned against God and against you. I am no longer fit to be called your son; treat me as one of your hired workers." So he got up and started back to his father.

He was still a long way from his home when his father saw him; his heart was filled with pity, and he ran, threw his arms around his son, and kissed him. "Father," the son said, "I have sinned against God and against you. I am no longer fit to be called your son."

But the father called to his servant. "Hurry!" he said. "Bring the best robe and put it on him. Put a ring on his finger and shoes on his feet. Then go and get the prize calf and kill it, and let us celebrate with a feast. For this son of mine was dead, but now he is alive; he was lost, but now he has been found."

*Luke 14:11-24*

* * *

We must come to love even our wounds.

Friedrich Nietzsche

* * *

Is my gloom, after all, Shade of His hand, out-stretched caressingly?

Francis Thompson in *The Hound of Heaven*

\* \* \*

A friend is someone who knows the song in your heart and sings it back to you when you forget how it goes.

\* \* \*

A man who is unable to despair has not need to be alive.

Johann Wolfgang von Goethe

\* \* \*

All despair is, in its deepest nature, despair of God's mercy, and you can hardly do worse.

Katherine Anne Porter

\* \* \*

The supreme greatness of Christianity derives from the fact that it does not seek a supernatural remedy against suffering, but a supernatural use for suffering.

Simone Weil

\* \* \*

Looking at what happened in Christ's life, Christians will expect to be saved, not from danger and suffering, but in danger and suffering.

Dorothy Sayers

\* \* \*

It is only in extreme situations that man becomes aware who he is.

Karl Jasper

* * *

In my misery it was revealed to me that man can come to that Heart only through the sense of separation from It which is called sin.

William Butler Yeats

* * *

Jesus also told this parable to people who were sure of their own goodness and despised everybody else:

"Once there were two men who went up to the Temple to pray: one was a Pharisee [religious partisan], the other a tax collector. The Pharisee stood apart by himself and prayed: 'I thank you, God, that I am not greedy, dishonest or an adulterer, like everybody else. I thank you that I am not like that tax collector over there. I fast two days a week, and give you one tenth of all my income.'

"But the tax collector stood at a distance and would not even raise his face to heaven, but beat on his breast and said: 'God, have pity on me, a sinner.'

"'I tell you," said Jesus, "the tax collector, and not the Pharisee, was the one who went home in God's good graces."

*Luke 18:9-13*

* * *

Heart's wave could not curl, nor beautifully break into the foam of spirit, did not the ageless, silent rock of destiny stand in its path.

Friedrich Holderlin

* * *

**48**

Happiness is more a matter of instants than of hours.

* * *

Behind tranquility often lies conquered unhappiness.

Eleanor Roosevelt

* * *

She moves fearlessly amid the most burning mysteries. She has life on her side. In harmless as well as in frightful matters, she recognizes one Force with many disguises — a Force which means to be generous, even when it causes death.

Rainer Maria Rilke on Lou Andreas-Salome

* * *

It is sometimes just at the moment when you think that everything is lost that the intimation arrives which may save you. You've knocked on all the doors which lead nowhere, and then you stumble without knowing in on the only door through which you can enter — which you might have sought in vain for a hundred years. And it opens of its own accord.

Marcel Proust in *Remembrance of Things Past*

* * *

Gerald and I will have our picnic. I am planning it now. Our many picnics. After I have traveled the tunnel and been welcomed into the light, I will search the faces for one of my favorite people, and he will be there. Gerald and I will walk together and laugh and embrace, sealed as friends forever through years of knowledge of how dearly we still loved each other after all the weeping was done.

And Whoever is in charge of all this will walk with us, and will help us to sort out the mysteries and help us to complete the healing. Walls will fall and we will see each other more clearly — all of us, the Mormons and the Catholics and the Jews and the Moslems and the straights and the gays and the blacks and the whites and the women and the men. Confusions will lift like fog from the Golden Gate Bridge on a good summer day.

Carol Lyn Pearson in Goodbye, I Love You

* * *

God will wipe away every tear from their eyes, and death shall be no more, nor grief, nor crying, nor pain.

Revelations 21:4

* * *

### A Story and a Poem for a Teacher with AIDS

The first time I visited him I didn't know he had AIDS. The door to his hospital room bore an infection warning, but the malady wasn't specified. Though he told me as chaplain that he was seriously ill he never used the heavy word.

His first stay was for about six weeks in the summer of 1984. He was in his early 30s, taught literature and directed plays in an out-of-town high school. We swapped stories about our teaching experiences, our favorite writers, our special books.

For his own protection he couldn't go back to teaching. So he lived with his family until he returned to the hospital this past March. As time dragged by, his eyes occasionally radiated a kind of frightened brightness. Once I tried to hold his hand, but he pulled away. "We didn't touch in our family."

One day in mid-June he suddenly blurted out: "I'm bored. Tell me a story." He had caught me by surprise, but I tried to think of a story that a lover of literature would like. Luckily, I thought of a true one of my own.

Fourteen summers ago I was visiting the Baltimore poet Josephine Jacobsen in her New Hamphire home. On the morning of my departure I discovered in my guest room a small book of her poems which had been published in 1940 by a small press in Texas. I hadn't been aware such a volume existed, and judged that it had been a limited edition that was now out of print. The title was *Let Each Man Remember*. I asked whether I might borrow it and was graciously told to accept it as a gift.

So I said goodbye and headed down the highway. Some hours later, as my lunch hungers surfaced, I saw a Howard Johnson's and thought of my favorite milky clam chowder. Parking my car, I decided to take my gift book with me.

Before long I was seated at the counter and gave my order to a young waitress. Then I began to read from the book which I thought I had rather inconspicuously opened on the counter.

Another teen-age waitress passed by and casually remarked: "That's a lovely book, isn't it?"

I couldn't believe that she was talking to me or that she had recognized the discolored volume in my hands. "You mean *this* book?"

"Yes," she answered brightly. "I discovered it last summer in an old bookshop in Maine. Each night at camp I read a different poem to the kids in my cabin. My favorite is one of the sonnets up front." She leaned over the book, flipped some pages, and announced: "Yes, there it is. I know it by heart."

I gazed increduously at that shining youngster, whose parents had probably been youngsters when this poem was published and who was now passionate with praise for these words by a stranger.

I told her I had just left the author of this book, left her standing on the steps of that "Winter Castle" which gave its name to the section of the book where the girl's favorite poem appeared.

Now it was the waitress's turn to stare in disbelief. To help convince her, I took her name and address and mailed them to the poet, who sent a loving letter to her youthful admirer...

My bored friend with AIDS had been listening intently. After I had finished he pursed his lips and held them that way for some thoughtful moments. Then, as a wry smile dismantled the pursing, he commented softly: "I guess there are good infections too."

Not long afterwards I came across that bridge-building book in my library. An impulse prompted me to turn to the title poem, "Let Each Man Remember:"

*There is a terrible hour in the early morning*
*When men awake and look on the day that brings*
*The hateful adventure, approaching with no less*
  *certainty*
*Than the light that grows, the untroubled bird that*
  *sings.*

*It does not matter what we have to consider:*
*Whether the difficult word, or the surgeon's knife,*
*The last silver goblet to pawn, or the fatal letter,*
*Or the prospect of going on with a particular life.*

*The point is, they rise; always they seem to have risen,*
*(They always will rise, I suppose), by courage alone.*
*Somehow, by this or that, they engender courage,*
*Courage bred in the flesh that is sick to the bone.*

*Each in his fashion, they compass their set intent*
*To rout the reluctant sword from the gripping*
  *sheath,*
*By thinking, perhaps, upon the Blessed Sacrament,*
*Or perhaps by coffee, or perhaps by gritted teeth.*

*It is indisputable that some turn solemn or savage,*

*While others have found that it serves them best*
  *to be glib*
*When they inwardly lean and listen, listen for*
  *courage,*
*That bitter and curious thing beneath the rib.*

*With nothing to gain, perhaps, and no sane reason*
*To put up a fight, they grip and hang by the thread*
*As fierce and still as a swinging threatened spider.*
*They are too brave to say, It is simpler to be dead.*

*Let each man remember, who opens his eyes to that*
  *morning,*
*How many men have braced him to meet the light,*
*And pious or ribald, one way or another, how many*
*Will smile in its face, when he is at peace in the night.*

Why hadn't I thought of it sooner? I had to show this
poem to my friend, who believed in good infections. So I
paid a hasty visit to his hospital room.

And discovered that his trials were over. But in my
heart's eye I could see him: in the midst of countless,
applaluding, illuminating smiles, Steve was at last at
peace.

Joseph Gallagher
*The Baltimore Evening Sun*: Sept. 4, 1985

\* \* \*

May He support us all the day long
till the shadows lengthen
and the evening comes
and the busy world is hushed
and the fever of life is over
and our work is done.

Then
in His mercy
may He give us a safe lodging
and a holy rest
and peace at the last.

John Henry Newman

If you would like a beautiful recording of Father Gallagher reading his letter to a friend with AIDS, please send your name and address and $7.95 plus $2.00 shipping and handling to: Credence Cassettes, Box 414291, Kansas City, MO 64141 or call toll free 1-800-821-7926. Use this number when ordering: AA2027, English; AA2030, Spanish.